A Healing System

Workbook

Compendium

Implementation - Arthritis - Quiz

By Stuart Farrel

ISBN-13: **978-1495327933**

Cover picture by Stuart and Elizabeth Farrel: **Rays of Hope with a Silver Lining**

We, the human race, have reached an auspicious time in our evolutionary process. **It happened in the last decade, when science documented the ideal diet.** It is now up to us, the general population, to absorb and embrace this knowledge. The implementation will eliminate or reduce five of the top seven killer diseases, and significantly reduce the onset of many more. Our government will not help us. Big corporations will not help us. Sadly, these two groups are part of the problem and will continue to stand against us. So, good health is up to us.

Stuart Farrel

Disclaimer

I am not a doctor, health care professional, or nutritionist. I've had no formal medical or nutritional training. Information presented in this book is from my personal experiences and the research of world renowned medical scientists.

What is presented in this compendium is derived from testing I've done on myself and family, plus extensive research in medical literature, and a great deal of experience, some of which is not presented.

The health information presented has not undergone clinical trials. Testimonials presented might be due to the placebo effect. I don't think so, but this is only my view.

Therefore, please do not use this compendium as a vehicle for self-diagnoses or treatment. Use this compendium as a guide to improve your judgment for long-term health care objectives. It is not a substitute for licensed health care. Do not use this book to treat any specific illness. No guarantee or assurance is specified or implied pertaining to specific results that may or may not be obtained.

If you are experiencing health problems, consult a licensed health care professional. The earlier disease detection happens, the better your chances for successful treatment.

Contents

Implementation Workbook

Arthritis Workbook

Quiz Workbook

A Healing System

Implementation Workbook

Introduction

This implementation workbook has been provided for those who have read the book **A HEALING SYSTEM** and have decided to transition into the lifestyle and dietary regimen suggested therein.

If nothing else, this book provides a flavor for the tasks involved in the transition process. Though detailed, please know that this book, with its set of transition-steps, is a suggested-process. The reader is encouraged to tailor it to meet their own needs.

Chapter 1: Preparation

This chapter provides the preparation tasks needed to help create a smooth transition to a healthier lifestyle. Schedule these tasks so that they are completed prior to the 'System Start Date' specified in Step 5 below. Once these are complete, they can be followed by the all-important transition tasks in Chapter 2.

Step 1—Make a Commitment

As with any new venture, success depends on commitment. A half-hearted attitude will only make the task more difficult. Change can be daunting, but only until new habit patterns are in place. Decide to get healthy no matter what it takes, and then get excited about the possibilities: healing, good health, more energy, improved thinking processes, and an upbeat attitude.

Step 2—Perform a Task Review

Do a thorough review of this entire workbook. Prepare your mind for the tasks to be performed, especially the 'discard' task, which might be psychologically uncomfortable.

Step 3—Train Your Support Team

Estimated Start Date _____

Identify and train your support group and staff of helpers. These are the people in your life who support what you are doing and have a vested interest in your success. They could be your best friend, family member, or spouse.

They will need to know—and probably be interested in—what you are about to do. Help them learn about the diet changes you will be making. Teach them about pH balancing and food combining. Talk with them about exercise plans you have or may want to create.

In short, build your team and get them involved, even if it is only one person—and especially if it is only one person. Also, there may be people in your life that won't be on the team but need to know something about the changes they will see, like drinking and diet modification. These people could be family members or individuals you live with who will not be part of your support group, like a younger sibling or infirmed grandparent. Maybe an infirmed grandparent is someone who could benefit from the healthier lifestyle as well.

How might you approach a potential team member? Phrases like this could get you started. "I've decided to get healthy and do it using information recently acquired. I'm thinking of it as a six week experiment involving diet, exercise, water intake, probiotics and more. Will you help me?" Tell him or her about your expectations for the program, the healing you are striving to achieve. Ask if he or she will be available to help you through the rough spots. If the person is agreeable and someone you want to talk with regularly, ask if he or she will work the remaining steps with you, even help you bring others onto your support team.

List the people you wish to talk to, and classify them as team members or simply individuals to be notified, write T or N in the space provided.

Name _____ **Team / Notify** ___ **Completion Date**
_____

Name _____ **Team / Notify** ___ **Completion Date**
_____

Name _____ **Team / Notify** ___ **Completion Date**
_____

Name _____ **Team / Notify** ___ **Completion Date**
_____

Name _____ **Team / Notify** ___ **Completion Date**
_____

Name _____ **Team / Notify** ___ **Completion Date**
_____

Name _____ **Team / Notify** ___ **Completion Date**
_____

Step 4—Establish a Schedule

Decide how much time to allow for the preparation tasks. I recommend at least a week. This may seem like a long time, but consider what is about to happen. The Task Review described above is important for the changes you are about to make and should not be rushed. Let the steps sink in and try to image what it will be like—not only the new lifestyle, but performing the steps and what they mean to your well-being. Also, sharing can be the most time-consuming part of any process, especially if it involves training people or sharing the training activities.

Space for estimated start times are provided with each step in the process so you can create a schedule. You probably noticed blank schedule fields when performing the Task Review in Step 2.

Step 5—Pick a '*System*' Start Date

Pick the day you plan to begin the new dietary regimen and lifestyle. My suggestion would be to pick a Saturday, especially if you work a normal workweek. This schedule also makes it more likely that your support group will be available for the launch, the first two days. All preliminary tasks must be completed by this date.

'*System*' Start Date _____

Also, write the start date in the space provided at the beginning of Chapter 2. Keep in mind that prior to starting, all preparation tasks must be complete—tasks like the review, people notification, and more.

Step 6—Copy and Post Documents

Estimated Posting Date _____

Copy these documents (seven pages) from the appendices and post them on the refrigerator and nearby cupboards. The documents are:

A. Quick reference sheets (3 pages)   **Date of posting** _____

B. Food combining chart (2 pages)   **Date of posting** _____

C. Grocery Starter-List   **Date of posting** _____

D. Task List   **Date of posting** _____

Step 7—Memorize Success Keys

Estimated Start Date _____

Memorize the suggested items from Chapter 5 of this workbook. Expect this step to take time.

Actual Start Date _____

Actual Completion Date _____

Step 8—Buy Recipe Books

Estimated Start Date _____

Buy books of recipes for your new dietary regimen. Two books with recipes that might be good for your library are *Prevent and Reverse Heart Disease* by Dr. Caldwell B. Esselstyn and *Forks Over Knives* by Gene Stone.

Book title _____ **Purchase Date** _____

Book title _____ **Purchase Date** _____

Book title _____ **Purchase Date** _____

Step 9—Review Recipes

Estimated Start Date _____

Review recipes from the books you have purchased. Perhaps make a list of those that interest you most, and modify others as needed.

Date of Final Review _____

Step 10—Create a One Week Menu

Estimated Start Date _____

Make a list of menu items for your first week on the new diet. As an aid, use the menu template from the appendix.

Date of Template Copy _____

With the template in hand, begin filling it out based on your recipes of choice from the books you previously purchased. Or, you can create your own recipes and use them in combination with those from the books.

This step is actually an ongoing task. Begin by identifying a starter-set of recipes and then expect to add and change them over the years.

Instead of printing the template, you could make a computer copy using your favorite word processing or spreadsheet program.

Actual Start Date _____

Actual Completion Date _____

Step 11—Make Two Grocery Lists

Estimated Start Date _____

The grocery list you are about to create is a valuable tool to use until you become familiar with the new food items, including which foods are legal and which are to be avoided.

Using the existing Grocery Starter List, add additional food items that you wish to have on hand. Now make a copy of the modified Grocery Starter List and simply name it Grocery List.

Identify food items present in your cupboards, refrigerator and freezer; determine if they are items to be disposed of or kept. Do this by placing a check mark on the Grocery List next to items that you already have in your cupboards, refrigerator or freezer. These are items that need not be purchased. When you go to the grocery store, these checked items can be ignored.

You now have two grocery lists:
- The modified Grocery Starter List mounted on your refrigerator.
- The Grocery List to be used at the store in a later step.

It is a good idea to maintain both lists, one for reference posted in plain sight, and one for trips to the grocery store. Eventually neither will be needed, but for now the two lists serve an important purpose, and that is to help you become quickly familiar with the new food items. It would be a good idea not to underestimate the importance of these two lists.

Step 12—Buy Probiotics

Estimated Start Date _____

Go to a health-food store and get a good probiotic[1]. Ask the staff for help if needed.

Item purchased _____ **Purchase Date** _____

Delay taking probiotics until the day after you begin the new dietary regimen. A separate step is provided for your probiotic start date.

Step 13—Work Toward Task List Completion

Estimated Start Date _____

Fill out the Task List copied from the appendix. Complete each preparation task prior to the Start Day. Events may occur that delay or impede your initial plan. Simply adjust the schedule as required. NOTE: It is important to keep the process stress free and enjoy the journey.

NOTES and PLANS

_____

_____

_____

_____

_____

_____

_____

_____

_____

_____

---

[1] Probiotics are used to balance gut flora, which is critical to human health. For details, see the Gut Flora sections in the book *A Healing System.*

Chapter 2: Day One

Check your task list. All preliminary tasks should have been previously completed. Today begins the first day of the rest of your healthy life.

Step 1—Begin the Hydration Regimen

Today begins the new drinking regimen.[2]

We must ingest liquids, and water is best, and at room temperature. Avoid drinks with corn syrup, carbonation, processed fructose, sugar, honey, guava, stevia, or alcohol.

Drink an average of five and a half ounces per hour. This estimate is based on a number of inputs, including my family physician and the Mayo Clinic. There are many factors that determine how much water is enough for a given person. These factors include, but are not limited to the following:

- Weight: Bigger means above average water consumption, and smaller means less
- Activity level: More active means above average water consumption, and less active means less water
- Time outdoors: Being outside more often than average increases the need for water
- Stress: A stressful lifestyle increases the need for water
- Pollution exposure: Pollution increases the need for water
- Cleansing: A person experiencing cleansing needs more water

A doctor told me that starting this regimen would keep me running to the bathroom, but only for a couple of months. This has been my experience.

Do drink a cup of water fifteen minutes before meals, and do not drink during or immediately after meals. Some people would rather not drink water. If this is you, try adding a few drops of fresh lemon juice. This does not mean make lemonade.

Sipping during a meal is not drinking. Nothing is black and white. Simply address the intent of the drinking rule.

---

[2] For details and an explanation, see the hydration sections of the book *A Healing System*.

Step 2—Have Breakfast

This could be your last unhealthy meal. Try not to enjoy it too much. Remember to drink water fifteen minutes prior to the meal, and then do not drink during or immediately after the meal.

Because you are new to the drinking regimen, you may feel the urge to drink during the meal. If the urge is too strong, then take a sip of water, but keep the volume as low as possible. The urge to sip may dissipate over time.

Step 3—Keep the Good Food

Give away or throw out your unhealthy groceries. Do not throw out items that were checked on the Grocery List.

Step 4—Buy Groceries

Buy groceries from your prepared Grocery List. Remember to take a writing implement with you to the store. Do not buy checked items. These are already in the pantry. At the grocery store, you might buy items that are not on the list. If so, add them to your list after placing them in the cart. The Grocery List, with the additional updates, will be used in a later step.

Step 5—Eat a Healthy Meal

Prepare and eat your first meal from your pantry or the groceries purchased. Use the menu previously created for this purpose. Remember to drink water fifteen minutes prior to the meal, and then do not drink during or immediately after the meal.

NOTES and PLANS

_____

_____

_____

_____

_____

_____

Chapter 3: Day Two

This is your first full day on the new regimen. Please remember to be patient with yourself. If you took my scheduling suggestion, then today is Sunday, a day of rest and relaxation. This is a great day to set a psychological tone for the week.

Start Probiotics

First thing in the morning, on an empty stomach, take your first probiotic capsule with plenty of water. Most probiotics recommend one capsule per day. This is the beginning of a daily regimen that will last at least a week.

Make a Schedule

This is not necessarily a schedule to be followed, although that is surely acceptable. The intent of making a schedule is to help you understand how to think about important timing considerations and issues that may arise. For instance, what activities may interfere with your new lifestyle, such as your children's soccer practice, the night-school class, or the vacation in two months? How will your meal preparation, hydration, or exercise schedule dovetail with family life? These are things to consider. There may be no significant impact. Even so, it is best to plan rather than adjust on the fly and under stress.

Create an Updated Grocery List

On your computer or manually, make a clean copy of the existing scribbled-on grocery list, and then post it on the refrigerator. Place the old copies in an archive folder.

NOTES and PLANS

_____

_____

_____

_____

_____

Chapter 4: Making Progress

Your first two days are complete and new habits have likely begun to replace the old. You may wish to document your progress, feelings, and complaints in a type of diary. Such a document can help surface issues that need to be addressed. Also share your thoughts and concerns with your support team. This may help improve the process and avert problems.

Review the Startup Experiences List

What you are likely to experience during start-up (the first few weeks) is well known to those of us who have already been through it. Here is a partial list.

    A. Dislike of some foods.

    B. Can't get the new spicing and flavoring quite right.

    C. Hunger.

    D. Difficulty scheduling drinking around meals and exercise.

    E. Impatience - waiting for tastes to change, for adaptation to the new diet.

    F. Being consistent with the exercise regimen.

Allow yourself time to adjust to the new regimen. It will probably take more than a week or two before you settle into this important new lifestyle. Be patient with yourself.

Think About Exercise

After a few days—whenever is comfortable—make and implement an exercise plan. Consider when you would like to exercise, how much exercise to start with, and when to increase it. Think about building it into your schedule. Use the following page to record your thoughts. It can take six weeks to get in shape. The older you are the longer it might take. Do not be in a hurry.

Exercise should generally be done three to five days a week. However there are maintenance exercises to be done daily. This is especially important for couch potatoes, the infirmed, or the elderly who get no other type of exercise. The book **A HEALING SYSTEM** discusses a maintenance exercise called the five rites taken from the book **ANCIENT SECRETS OF THE FOUNTAIN OF YOUTH** by Peter Kelder. You may wish to consider it.

NOTES and PLANS

Chapter 5: Memorization

Here are eight items, that if memorized, will smooth the implementation path. The concepts are important. The wording is not. So there is no need to memorize the exact phrasing of these items.

1. Have a clear understanding of the phrases **alkaline producing** and **acid producing** foods.

2. Drink **five point five ounces of water every hour** during the healing process.

3. Drink a cup of **water fifteen minutes before** meals and take **no liquids during or immediately after** eating.

4. Some citrus is **acid in** and **alkali out**.

5. **Legumes, dried beans, almonds**, plus **sesame and hemp seeds** are protein and yet have an **alkaline effect** on the body.

6. Neither **melon** nor **citrus** should be combined with any other foods, or each other. Some **fruits can be eaten together**, but cannot be combined with other foods, such as proteins, starches or carbohydrates. Sweet fruits (a category of fruit) should not be eaten with non-sweet fruits.

7. **Do not mix proteins with carbohydrates**.

8. Exercise is important, and so is the **right amount of exercise**. Do not over exercise.

NOTES and PLANS

_____

_____

_____

_____

_____

Appendix: Quick Reference Sheet 1

Key Points to Remember

Attitude is Everything

What we think and believe will determine how, when, and if we heal. Remember the placebo and nocebo effects.

PH Balancing

Eat 30 percent or less acid producing foods (generally proteins) daily.

Eat 70 percent or more alkali producing foods (generally fruits and vegetables) daily.

Foods you might think are acid producing but are actually alkali producing:
    Almonds, beans, oranges, lemons, and the seeds hemp and sesame.

Food Combining

Combine vegetables with only one of protein or carbohydrates.

Eat these by themselves: citrus, melons, and sweet fruits.

Exercise

Exercise for waste removal and vital organ massage.

Do not over exercise.

With a degenerative disease, do only mild stretching and deep breathing.

Do not exercise too close to meals.

Drinking

Drink fifteen minutes before meals.

Drink five point five ounces of water per hour

Do not drink during meals.

Do not drink for a minimum of twenty to thirty minutes after meals.

Between Meals

Wait about three hours after a meal before ingesting another meal.

Plant-Based Whole Foods

Our diet should consist only of non-GMO, oil-free, plant-based whole foods. Eat foods that are as close to nature as possible. Do not eat processed foods, or any substance that had a mother.

Probiotics

Start the new dietary regimen by balancing gut flora.

Genetically Engineered Foods

Children should avoid GMOs because children are more susceptible to the problems caused by cross splicing gene species into our food. Their immune systems are immature. Adults should avoid them because of the potential health hazards.

Appendix: Quick Reference Sheet 2

ACID Producing Food Chart

These foods should be 30 percent or less of daily intake.

Apricot	Coffee	Molasses	Red Currant
Banana, Ripe	Cranberry	Mustard	Rice
Barley	Currant	Oats	Squash, winter
Barley Malt Syrup	Date	Orange	Strawberry
Beet Sugar	Grains	Papaya	Sunflower seeds
Black Currant	Grapes	Pasta	Tangerine
Blueberry	Grapefruit	Peach	Tea (Black)
Brown Rice	Hazelnuts	Peanut	Vinegar
Brown Rice Syrup	Honey	Pear	Walnuts
Cantaloupe	Italian Plum	Peas	Watermelon
Carob	Lentils	Pistachios	Wheat
Cashews	Macadamia Nuts	Plums *	White Sugar
Cherry, Sweet	Mandarin Orange	Prunes *	Wine
Chocolate	Mango	Raspberry	

* These foods leave an alkaline ash but have an acidifying effect on the body.

The following foods leave a neutral ash but have an acidifying effect on the body:
corn oil, corn syrup, sugar (refined) and olive oil.

ALKALI Producing Food Chart

These foods should be 70 percent or more of daily intake.

Alfalfa grass	Celery	Lettuce	Raisins
Almonds (sparingly)	Chard	Lima beans	Raspberries
Apples	Cherries, sour	Limes	Rhubarb *
Apricots	Chives	Millet	Rutabaga
Asparagus	Coconut	Molasses	Sauerkraut *
Avocado (fat & protein)	Cucumber	Mushrooms	Sesame seeds
Bananas	Dates, dried	Muskmelon	Soy *
Beans, dried	Fig, dried	Onions	Spelt
Beet greens	Garlic	Oranges	Spinach
Beets	Grapes	Parsnips	Strawberries
Blackberries	Green beans	Peaches	Tangerines
Brazil nuts (sparingly)	Hemp seeds	Pears	Tofu *
Broccoli	Kohlrabi	Peas	Tomatoes
Brussels sprouts	Leeks (bulbs)	Pineapple	Turnip
Cabbage	Lemons	Potatoes	Watermelon
Carrot	Lentils	Radish	Zucchini
Cauliflower			

* Not recommended—Leave an alkaline ash; however, they have other properties that are detrimental to the body.

Appendix - Quick Reference Sheet 3

Overview - Health Improvement Guide

If you have one of the following, your problem may be solved with **pH balancing** alone. Try cutting back significantly on acid-producing foods.

- Arthritis
- Fibromyalgia
- Gallbladder problems
- Diabetes I or II
- Hemorrhoids
- Kidney infections
- Osteoporosis

If you have a serious disease, then you probably need more than pH balancing. Try a **nutritious, non-GMO, oil-free, plant-based whole foods** diet plus **pH balancing, trophology**, and proper *careful* **exercise**, including deep breathing and stretching. This advice pertains to diseases such as the following:

- Cancer
- Multiple Sclerosis
- Diabetes I or II
- Cardiovascular disease
- Heart disease
- Alzheimer's

Start With Probiotics

When starting this or any new health regimen, begin with probiotics. If your gut is not healthy, you will not be healthy. With an unbalanced gut, healing will be more difficult if not impossible.

Avoid U.S. Commercial GMO Crops

Soy
Corn
Canola
Cotton
Sugar beets
Yellow squash
Zucchini
Papaya

Appendix: Food Combining Chart

When selecting foods for a meal, only include those that combine GOOD or EXCELLENT according to the chart below. Super scripts apply to numbered notes following the chart.

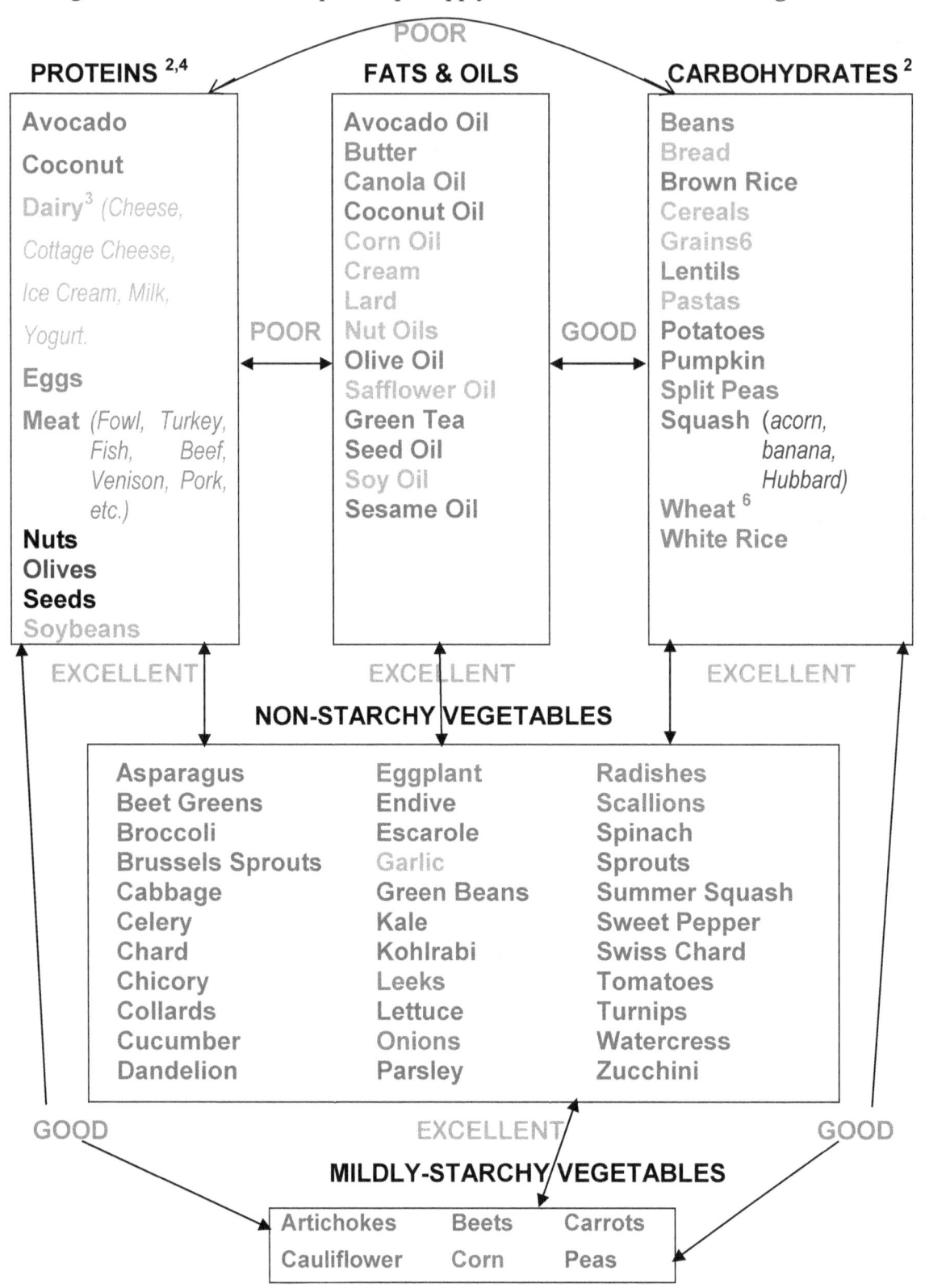

POOR

PROTEINS [2,4]

Avocado
Coconut
Dairy[3] *(Cheese,*
Cottage Cheese,
Ice Cream, Milk,
Yogurt.
Eggs
Meat *(Fowl, Turkey,*
Fish, Beef,
Venison, Pork,
etc.)
Nuts
Olives
Seeds
Soybeans

FATS & OILS

Avocado Oil
Butter
Canola Oil
Coconut Oil
Corn Oil
Cream
Lard
Nut Oils
Olive Oil
Safflower Oil
Green Tea
Seed Oil
Soy Oil
Sesame Oil

CARBOHYDRATES [2]

Beans
Bread
Brown Rice
Cereals
Grains6
Lentils
Pastas
Potatoes
Pumpkin
Split Peas
Squash *(acorn,*
banana,
Hubbard)
Wheat [6]
White Rice

POOR ⟷ **GOOD**

EXCELLENT   **EXCELLENT**   **EXCELLENT**

NON-STARCHY VEGETABLES

Asparagus	Eggplant	Radishes
Beet Greens	Endive	Scallions
Broccoli	Escarole	Spinach
Brussels Sprouts	Garlic	Sprouts
Cabbage	Green Beans	Summer Squash
Celery	Kale	Sweet Pepper
Chard	Kohlrabi	Swiss Chard
Chicory	Leeks	Tomatoes
Collards	Lettuce	Turnips
Cucumber	Onions	Watercress
Dandelion	Parsley	Zucchini

GOOD   **EXCELLENT**   **GOOD**

MILDLY-STARCHY VEGETABLES

Artichokes	Beets	Carrots
Cauliflower	Corn	Peas

Food Combining Chart (Continued)

ACID FRUIT	SUB-ACID FRUIT	SWEET FRUIT	MELON
Blackberry	Apple	Bananas	Cantaloupe
Grapefruit	Apricot	Dates	Casaba
Lemon/Lime	Blueberry	Currants	Crenshaw
Orange	Cherry	Figs	Honeydew
Pineapple	Kiwi	Grapes	Persian
Plum (sour)	Mango	Papaya	Watermelon
Pomegranate	Peach	Persimmon	
Raspberry	Pear	Prunes	
Sour Apple	Plum (sweet)	Raisins	
Strawberry			

FRUITS are best when eaten alone or as a meal such as breakfast when the stomach is empty of other foods. Each fruit-group should be eaten separately from other fruit-groups, especially melons and sweet fruits.

NOTES

1. Also refer to alkali and acid foods chart.

2. Food combining is also effective in curing some bowel disorders.

3. Carbohydrates and proteins should never be eaten together, or during the same meal period.

4. Milk and other dairy products are discouraged for human consumption *(Exception: mother's breast milk is highly recommended for babies of the same species.)*

5. Concentrated proteins are unnecessary. Use as a condiment, not as a main course. In any case, eat no more than one each meal.

6. Garlic has been reported to produce adverse side effects, and should be considered for medicinal use only.

7. Good when sprouted to vegetable state before consumption.

8. *"All things in moderation, including moderation."* Socrates

9. Corn, although a grain, is placed in the mildly starchy vegetables category because that is how it behaves. Use only non-GMO corn and its 50 plus by-products.

WARNING The following crops are genetically modified in the United States: Soy, Corn, Sugar beets, Cotton, Canola, Hawaiian papaya, Zucchini and Yellow squash.

The source for this chart comes from the following web-page:
http://www.AHealingSystem.com/foodcombining.html

Appendix: AHS Grocery Starter-List

Buy fresh and organic whenever possible.

Fruit	Salad	Legumes	Vegetables	Nuts, Raw
Apple *	Avocado @	Beans, dried *	Acorn squash	Almonds * @
Cantaloupe *	Bell peppers	Chickpeas *	Asparagus	Brazil nuts @
Honeydew *	Carrots	Lentils *	Broccoli *	Walnuts @
Kiwi *	Celery *	Lima beans *	Eggplant	
Orange *	Cucumber	Peas, fresh *	Green beans	
	Kale *	Split peas *	Spaghetti squash	
	Lettuce *		String beans	
	Pepperoncini		Sugar snap peas	
	Spinach *		Sweet potatoes *	
	Sprouts			

Grains	Liquids	Seeds	Meals
Amaranth	Apple juice	Chia	Amy's (no cheese) dinners
Barley	Carrot juice	Flax (ground)	Grits #
Millet	Distilled H_2O	Hemp	Japanese vegetable makkis
Quinoa	Oat milk	Pine nuts	Oatmeal
Rice, brown	Orange juice	Pumpkin	Roasted vegetables
	Rice milk	Sesame *	Soup
		Sunflower	Steamed vegetables

Other	Herbs	Condiments	Supplements
Bread, sprouted	Basil	Bragg Liquid Protein	Kelp (iodine) *
Herbal teas	Cinnamon	Honey	Probiotics
Shredded wheat	Garlic	Iodized sea salt	Vitamin B12
Vegetable broth	Ginger	Pepper	Vitamin D_2
	Parsley	Poultry seasoning	

* These foods are alkaline ash and may contains alkaline buffering elements.

@ These foods are high in fats so use sparingly. Heart disease patients should avoid these foods.

\# WARNING: In the United States, this food may be genetically modified because it is corn.

Soy products are missing for two reasons: they are genetically modified in the United States, plus soy is the most mucus forming (slightly toxic) plant humans ingest.

Appendix: Task List

Note that there are underline areas for making check marks or Xs to indicate completion.

PREPARATION

1. __ Review the entire Implementation Workbook, working toward an understanding of what is involved. This can help eliminate surprises and stress.

2. __ Identify, train, and notify support people and family.

3. __ Pick a start date for system implementation.

      The date: _____

4. __ Copy and post the six documents.

5. __ Memorize success keys.

6. __ Buy and review recipe books.

7. __ Create a one week menu using the template provided.

8. __ Make two grocery lists.

9. __ Buy probiotics.

DAY ONE
START DATE _____

1. __ Start hydrating

2. __ Breakfast

3. __ Keep the good food and remove the rest

4. __ Buy groceries

5. __ Eat your first healthy meal

DAY TWO

1. __ Start probiotics first thing in the morning on an empty stomach with plenty of water.

2. __ Make a schedule. Think about how your new lifestyle will dovetail with existing daily routines.

3. __ Create an updated grocery list from the scribbled-on list used at the grocery store.

AFTER A FEW DAYS

__ Make an exercise plan. Decide how to begin, when to make increases and adjustments, list anyone who will exercise with you, and create a schedule. Now that a plan is available, you are ready to begin. Tomorrow is not too late.

Appendix: AHS Menu Template

The sample two day menu below demonstrates how to fill out the Weekly Menu template provided in the next appendix.

Symbols used: **B** - Breakfast, **L** - Lunch, **D** - Dinner. or M_1, M_2, M_3, M_4, where M = Meal.

Day	Recipe Name	Food Items Included	pH Type	Preparation Time	Comments
1 B	Oatmeal with Nuts	Oatmeal (not instant), almonds (less than 12), honey (minimal amount)	Acid	1 hour	A bit heavy for breakfast, but what most people are used to.
1 L	Salad and Seeds	Fresh mixed baby greens, green pepper, scallions, carrots, fresh spinach, tomatillo, yellow squash, zucchini, cucumber, celery, tomato, flax seeds (ground), sunflower seeds, pumpkin seeds, hemp seeds, sesame seeds, and a dressing of salt, pepper, ginger, water, and lemon juice	Mixed	15 minutes	Seed volume will determine just how filling the meal will be. Suggested starter amount for seeds would be a teaspoon of each. Ground flax seeds are sold as flax meal.

1 D	Steamed Vegetables	Some or all of the following: steamed asparagus, green beans, sugar snap peas, yams, broccoli, cauliflower, spices	Base	30 minutes	It is hard to get simpler than this.
1 D	Simple Dinner Salad	Fresh spinach, butter lettuce, celery, avocado, broccoli flowers, sunflower seeds, and a dressing of garlic, salt, water, and lemon juice	Mixed	10 minutes	
2 B	Kiwi and Apple	One kiwi and one organic Fuji apple	Base	10 seconds	If more volume is need, double the dose.
2 L	Potatoes au Simple	Diced steamed sweet potato, yellow potato, yellow onion, and split peas (pre-cooked), raw diced tomatillo, vegetable broth, spices	Base	30 minutes	A quick, simple and tasty alkaline carbohydrate meal with protein (split pees).
2 D	Vegetable Makkis	Nori, Sushi rice, carrots, cucumber, assorted hydrated seaweeds, avocado, wasabi, pickled ginger, Bragg's liquid protein or soy sauce	Mixed	1 hour	This simple meal takes practice to make properly; especially making the sticky rice.

2 D	Large Dinner Salad	Mixed baby greens, green pepper, scallions, carrots, fresh spinach, tomatillo, yellow squash, cucumber, celery, tomato, sprouts, dressing of salt, pepper, basil, water, lime juice	Mixed	10 minutes	Simple and healthy, and the dressing can be made in the salad bowl without pre-mixing.

Appendix: AHS Weekly Menu

Fill out this template to produce a life-healthy weekly menu. The blank second page should be duplicated as many times as required.

Symbols used: **B** - Breakfast, **L** - Lunch, **D** - Dinner. or M_1, M_2, M_3, M_4, where M = Meal.

Day & Meal	Recipe Name	Food Items Included	pH Type	Preparation Time	Comments

If you have questions, communicate with us via the Contact Us web page of the website below. Please place 'AHS Implementation Workbook' on the subject line.

www.AHealthSystem.com

A Healing System

Arthritis

Workbook

Introduction

This workbook has been prepared to help readers aggressively reverse their arthritis. It is a subset of the book **A HEALING SYSTEM**, which should be read first to gain a complete understanding of the what and why involved.

If nothing else, this workbook gives readers a flavor for the tasks this author believes are necessary to facilitate arthritis reversal in the shortest possible timeframe. It has worked for the author and his friends.

Implementing every suggested action is a daunting task. Therefore the actions suggested are presented in order of importance, *for arthritis sufferers who eat the Standard American Diet (SAD)*, which may be contributing to their discomfort.

Should you wish to implement the minimal subset of the actions presented, then use only the first action listed, restricting acid intake. In general, this simply means increasing fruits and vegetables and decreasing protein intake. Simple is good, but nothing is black and white. Tables are provided in the appendix for those who wish to be more rigorous during the acid-balancing process.

Warning: The diet suggested here might seem extreme. It is actually very moderate, sensible, and has been shown to be important in reducing arthritis symptoms plus improving general health. However, in most arthritis cases, it needs only be followed for 6 to 8 weeks. Most people have reported significant reversal within this timeframe.

Note to readers: The regimen presented in this book has worked for me and others. That does not mean it will work for you. However, this workbook exists because I believe it might work for you. This regimen has not been clinically test, which is expensive and needed. Maybe someday it will happen.

Only the human immune system and the placebo effect can heal the body.

The following four graphics are used in this workbook to indicate the content identified below each symbol.

         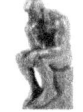

   Key Concept   Duration   Be careful   Reasoning

Chapter 1: Arthritis Reversal Overview

This chapter provides an overview of the considerations involved in the potential reversal of arthritis. For a more complete understanding of arthritis reversal and related body chemistry, see the book **A HEALING SYSTEM** which explains why the system might work, the body chemistry involved, plus it lists possible reasons people might find it difficult to address their problems.

Please note that arthritis seems to be an acidosis related disease. Therefore, this same workbook may also be helpful in reversing other acidosis related diseases like osteoporosis, gallbladder problems, stiff joints, and more.

The short-term lifestyle changes needed to reverse arthritis vary depending on arthritic severity. Someone who is severely crippled, perhaps in a wheelchair, will need a very different beginning than those who are fully functional.

Writing for everyone, in all the different debilitating arthritic states, is just not practical. Hopefully, this approach and the information provided will be adequate for any patient to glean their specific set of healing steps.

The following definitions will be important for readers to grasp the most critical action in arthritis reversal, pH balancing.

Acid	Having a pH below 7.0.
Acidic ash food	Foods whose digestion residue, or ash, has a pH below 7.0: acidic.
Alkali	Having a pH above 7.0. A common synonym is base.
Alkaline ash food	Foods whose digestion residue, or ash, has a pH above 7.0: alkaline.
Ash	The metabolic residue left after food has been digested and assimilated, also known as post-digestion ash.

The Reversal Process

There exists a set of seven important actions in the process of reversing arthritis.

Implement only that with which you can cope.

Please take your time absorbing this material. Reading it a few times can be helpful. Get help with anything you do not understand.

No matter the patient's state of dysfunction and pain, the same critical set of actions is needed to aggressively attack arthritis. These actions are presented in order of their importance. You may implement one action or more than one action, and you may stagger implementation, which means implementing the first action and then later adding the second, and so forth. Do what is most comfortable for you and your circumstances. Make it a fun experience. You have nothing to lose but your pain.

Arthritis Healing and Painkillers

Patients on painkillers should continue with them as needed. Hopefully the need will be gone after a few weeks—three to eight depending on the number of actions implemented.

Chapter 2: Arthritis Reversal Details

This chapter provides the what, why, how, and duration for each action item. They range in duration from one week to successful reversal. Each of you must determine what you can deal with and when to implement your selected actions.

1—Restrict Acid Ingestion

This is the most important action one can take to aid the reversal of arthritis.

Each day eat less than 30 percent from the acid producing food list and therefore more than 70 percent from the alkali producing food list. Lists are found in the appendix.

DO NOT EAT ONLY ALKALI PRODUCING FOODS. First, the body will become too alkaline and then it will hurt to urinate. Second, to heal, the body needs what is provided by both alkali and acid producing foods.

Continue until you are satisfied with the degree of reversal, and possibly longer.

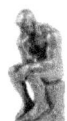

Restricting acid is the key, and is really about strictly controlling metabolic acidosis. This action, more than any other, facilitates arthritis reversal. So if you can only take one action, then take this one.

It may be possible to succeed by only restricting acid. Actions like exercise, probiotics, the healing-enhancement diet and hydration are support for the critical function of balancing acid intake.

The two acid-balancing food groups roughly break down as follows:

Acid   grains, seeds, nuts, pasta, bread

Alkali   vegetables, legumes and fruits

There are exceptions to each rule. See the two food lists in the appendix for more detail.

When looking at the food lists, please note that some items will defy common sense. For instance, an orange is acid on the plate, but alkali after the digestive process. See the book *A HEALING SYSTEM* for an explanation.

STRONG SUGGESTION: Eat **only alkali producing foods for the first two days**, but not for longer than that. After those two days, make acid foods 20 percent of daily faire, and increase the percentage slowly to 25 or 30 percent over a four-week timeframe.

RESTRICTING-ACID NOTES

Take a moment to note down foods from each of the two lists, foods you have, or foods you would like to have. Perhaps plan a few meals.

_____

_____

_____

_____

_____

_____

_____

_____

_____

_____

_____

2—Healing-Enhancement Diet

 Eat the ideal diet which is plant-based whole-foods, the healthiest diet known to science.

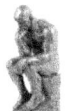 **The largest study of diet every conducted, "THE CHINA STUDY", involved over one hundred thousand people. It proved conclusively that a plant-based whole-food diet is the healthiest diet known to science. This means eating nonprocessed foods and no animal products, especially dairy. This diet is very basic and contains only fresh or frozen fruits, vegetables, legumes, nuts, seeds and grains like corn, rice, amaranth, quinoa, and millet.**

 Continue until you are satisfied with the degree of reversal.

A plant-based, whole-food diet will mean a significant change for most people. The change can be temporary. An appendix entitled *'Grocery List'* is provided to help orient readers toward the non-animal diet, foods that can be found in the fresh or frozen sections of most grocery stores.

DIET CHANGE NOTES

Take a moment to note down the foods you wish to purchase, where they might be found, and quantities to acquire. Also note foods in your cupboard or refrigerator that must be thrown out or given away because they will not be consumed and will likely go bad during the next 6 to 8 weeks.

_____

_____

_____

_____

_____

_____

3—Immune System Enhancement

 Avoid those foods that might aggravate healing.

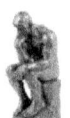 **Immune system enhancement is needed to ensure that no additional problems are presented to the body during the reversal process. This will ensure that the body's immune system is working primarily on the arthritis.**

 Continue until you are satisfied with the degree of reversal.

Since only our immune system can heal us, it is best to do whatever we can to enhance its ability to do the job. Diet is the primary and most critical ingredient in immune system health. Therefore only health-giving substances should be ingested. To that end, the substances listed below are either **unhealthy or negatively impact the body's immune system**, and therefore are not optimal for healing.

Genetically Modified Foods (GMOs)

Reasoning: Genetically Modifies Organisms (GMOs) are known immune system stressors. The health risks are simply not worth the gamble. Please see the appendix entitled *'Corn Warning'*. Know that this warning also applies to corn by-products plus soy and its by-products.

 DO NOT EAT GENETICALLY MODIFIED FOODS. These foods have had no long term human safety studies. Some are banned in over twenty countries. Children may be at greater risk because of their underdeveloped immune systems.

Desserts

Reasoning: These substances include candy, soda, sweets, or sugar of any kind; i.e., Baskin Robbins, the Yogurt Hut, the ice cream truck, bakeries, etc.

Oil and Foods Fried in Oil

Reasoning: These substances are either too fatty or contain sugar, plus can be difficult to digest, which means a stress on the body; chemically and energetically.

Dairy

Reasoning: The majority of the population is allergic to dairy at some level. Eating melted cheese is like trying to digest leather (stressful). These foods include, milk, cheese, butter, yogurt, kefir, and more.

Unhealthy Drinks

Reasoning: These substances are known immune system stressors: coffee, milk, tea, alcohol, chai, hot chocolate, and anything with a sweetener or carbonation.

Sweeteners

Reasoning: Sweeteners are mostly empty calories and innervate the body. They are neutral (not acid), but the innervation they cause creates an acidic condition.

Spices

Reasoning: Spices are a stressor to the immune system. Try to use only sea salt (iodized) and maybe a little pepper. It is best to stay away from highly spiced foods—hot or otherwise—at least until health returns.

Vinegar and Oil

Reasoning: Vinegar is acetic acid, not good for humans. Try a little fresh lemon juice instead of a regular salad dressing.

Smoking

Reasoning: Smoking of any kind is a stressor on the lungs and immune system.

Alcohol

Reasoning: Alcoholic drinks and foods are liver-related immune system stressors.

Dairy, Red Meat and Soy

Reasoning: These are the three most mucus forming foods, listed in order of severity (worst first), which means that they are toxic to the body at some level.

IMMUNE SYSTEM ENHANCEMENT NOTES

Take a moment to note down substances that will be difficult to avoid and suggest ways to do so.

_____

_____

_____

_____

_____

_____

_____

_____

_____

_____

_____

_____

_____

_____

_____

_____

4—Hydration

 Drink a minimum of five point five ounces of water per hour.

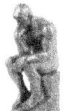 **Hydration (water) and exercise are needed by the body to remove cellular waste, unwanted substances, and toxins. The exercise pumps and the water flushes. Water is the removal medium. Soda pop is not a good removal medium.**

 Continue until you are satisfied with the degree of reversal, and then forever.

Bigger, more active people who work outdoors should consider six or more ounces per hour. The reverse is also true. People who are small in stature, slight of build, and sedentary may consume less than five ounces per hour, but probably not less than four ounces per hour.

An increase in liquid consumption for most people will increase bathroom frequency, but not forever. The number of trips per day will drop off after about eight weeks.

Although the reversal plan is for a few weeks only, the consumption requirement should be carried on as described in *A HEALING SYSTEM* for the rest of your life. Hydration is an important health consideration.

It is health giving to schedule meal consumption for fifteen minutes after drinking the hourly dose.

Acquire a water bottle and carry it everywhere you go. People who do not carry a water bottle are probably not adequately hydrated.

HYDRATION NOTES

Take a moment to note down plans and suggestions you may have for a water bottle and a system for remembering to drink each hour and 15 minutes before meals.

_____

_____

_____

_____

_____

_____

_____

_____

_____

_____

_____

_____

_____

_____

_____

5—Exercise

 Exercise properly every day to pump the lymphatic system.

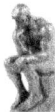 **Exercise and water are needed by the body to remove cellular waste, unwanted substances, and toxins. Exercise pumps the lymphatic system, and water flushes substances from it.**

 Continue until you are satisfied with the degree of reversal, and then forever.

Consider when you would like to exercise, how much exercise to start with, and when to increase it. Build it into your schedule.

If you are infirmed, then work out a simple stretching regimen that involves deep breathing. Deep breathing is important because it is the single most effective way of pumping the lymphatic system, though not adequate by itself. Muscle movement is the other half of the equation. Both are important.

Exercise should generally be done three to five days a week. However there is something called maintenance exercise that is done every day. This is important for couch potatoes, the infirmed, or the elderly who get no other type of exercise. The book *A HEALING SYSTEM* discusses a maintenance exercise I'm fond of called the Five Rites[3]. You may wish to consider it. It is the best ten minutes of my day.

First and for most, if you do nothing else, do this: ten **deep breaths** four times per day.

Second, **stretch** as many muscles as you can. Spend about ten minutes stretching each day.

Thirdly, **walk**, as briskly as you can. Try to walk for at least twenty minutes.

Fourth, the ideal is to perform twenty minutes or more of **aerobic exercise**. There are three primary types that give the best overall workout, in order of preference: running, swimming, or cycling. The intent is to get the heart

---

[3] *ANCIENT SECRETS OF THE FOUNTAIN OF YOUTH* by Peter Kelder

and breathing rates up and perhaps even generate some sweat. Do one of these three to five times per week if you can.

The Five Rites previously mentioned include deep breathing and stretching, as well as muscle-tone development.

Always do deep breathing and stretching. If some type of aerobic exercise is not possible, then try to walk. Whatever your condition or conditioning, do the best you can. Over time, whatever you are doing will get easier.

 If exercise is new to you, then start slowly and get help from someone who knows what they are doing. Before starting any exercise regimen, contact your doctor and tell him or her your plan. He can provide guidance relating your physical condition to the type and amount of exercise to be undertaken.

Although the reversal plan is for a few weeks only, exercise should be carried on as described in *A HEALING SYSTEM* for the rest of your life.

 If it hurts, do not do it. Too much enthusiasm can make us overdo. Be cautious. Give the body time to adjust—especially the connective tissue, which takes longer than muscles to adapt to increased physical stress.

EXERCISE NOTES

Take a moment to note down your proposed, or initial, exercise regimen.
Also create an exercise schedule. First thing in the morning is often best.

_____

_____

_____

_____

_____

_____

_____

6—Balance Intestinal Flora

 Take probiotics for a minimum of one week.

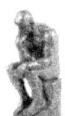 **Probiotics will balance intestinal flora which is the heart of the human immune system.**

Balance intestinal flora with probiotics, available at any health food store. Ask the store clerk for a reasonably priced probiotic from the refrigeration section. Follow directions on the bottle. Most probiotics are taken once per day. I prefer first thing in the morning, on an empty stomach, with plenty of water. Eighty three percent of the human immune system is in the gut wall, so balancing gut flora is important to the healing process. Try taking the probiotic for one week (minimum), beginning when the new dietary regimen is implemented.

 One week, minimum.

INTESTINAL FLORA NOTES

Take a moment to note down the stores where you might find probiotics, the day on which to make the trip, and the date to start taking them.

_____

_____

_____

_____

_____

_____

_____

_____

_____

7—Support Group

 Involve your support group.

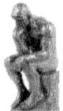 **The healing task is usually easier to perform when a support group is involved. Tell your friends what you are attempting and ask for their support. Share your experience with them throughout the reversal process. Friends help friends.**

 Continue until you are satisfied with the degree of reversal.

A support group can be a best friend, spouse, significant other, parent or caregiver, or a collection of all of these.

Food is the primary reversal tool in your arsenal. Therefore, if someone cooks for you, they could be your primary support person. Share your plans with them early in the process.

One excellent support option would be to find a friend willing to go through the healing process with you, someone else with arthritis who would also like to reverse their disease.

SUPPORT GROUP NOTES

Take a moment to note down the people in your support group. You could check off their names after each of them is brought up to date on your plans.

_____

_____

_____

_____

_____

_____

Chapter 3: Implementation Suggestions

There is work involved in preparing your mind and kitchen for a two-month lifestyle change. Here are some thoughts that might be helpful.

Change is not easy for most people. It can be less difficult when the mind accepts what must be done, when compliance is not malicious, and commitment abounds.

Take some time, prior to implementation, to review what is about to happen. Think about how you feel about it. Think about the goal—no pain. Obstacles are what we see when we do not focus on the goal.

Get help. Tap your support group. Talk with others who have been through the process. Find out what they struggled with and how they dealt with issues that arose.

Work to accept that some of the new foods will not taste as you would like. Experiment with new recipes. Never give up.

Exercise with caution. Give your body time to adapt to the new physical program. The goal is not to do everything you would like to do on the first day. The goal is to *work at getting to that point* where you can perform as you would like to perform.

In the kitchen, find an organization that facilitates the new food preparation activities. Perhaps there are tools needed to prepare fresh vegetables that you should make more easily accessible. Do you have a steamer? Maybe it should be out on the counter or stove for regular use. Think about helpful changes, and then experiment. If at first you don't succeed, try, try again. Enjoy the process of figuring out what works best for you.

Liquid Suggestion

1. Go to the kitchen and get a half-cup measuring cup.
2. Fill it to overflowing with water.
3. Drink it.
4. Set the kitchen timer for sixty minutes.
5. When the timer goes off, repeat these steps—all day long.

Chapter 4: Review

This chapter is a review of the actions that facilitate arthritis reversal. They are in no particular order.

A. Immediately start drinking five point five ounces of water per hour.

B. Talk to your support group about your arthritis reversal plan. Better yet, get a friend to do it along with you.

C. When beginning the new diet, simultaneously start a one-week (minimum) probiotic regimen.

D. Review and start your exercise plan. Exercise some each day.

E. Make a copy of and enhance the grocery list provided. Plan a few meals. Shop for needed groceries.

F. Eat a very basic diet that contains only fresh or frozen fruits, vegetables, legumes, nuts, seeds and grains such as corn, rice, amaranth, quinoa, and millet. Avoid the taboo substances, which includes GMOs and oils.

G. Keep your acid food consumption to less than 30 percent of daily intake, measured by either volume or weight (be consistent). Eye-balling quantity is usually good enough. Track acid consumption in writing—at least initially—to help you remember what is needed for the next meal. For instance, if your first two meals of the day were alkaline only, then the third and last meal could contain acid.

H. If possible, eat only alkali producing foods for the first two days, and then gradually increase acid the producing foods, but staying under 30 percent per day.

Here is one last thought. Fats have been linked to arthritis. Keep fats to a minimum. A low-fat diet, by today's standards, is too much fat. Less than three grams per meal would be ideal, but probably impossible to achieve. When the pain is gone and exercise is regular, then fats are less of a problem.

Appendix: Corn Warning

88% of U.S.A. corn crops are Genetically Modified (GM)

*** Children Should Avoid GM Products ***

There are 2 Types of GM Corn

1. BT corn

Each kernel has proteins that create the insecticide BT, which kills bugs who eat the corn, causing their abdomens to break open.

2. Roundup ready corn

Each kernel has proteins that create Roundup, the plant killer. Mothers, do you want your children Roundup Ready?

Potential GMO Corn Health Problems

- Digestive disorders
- Infertility problems in women
- Rashes
- Food allergies
- Autism in children
- and more

Children are at Greater Risk

Children have an immature immune system, and therefore are more susceptible to the health risks of genetically modified foods.

See the movie **GENETIC ROULETTE** or read the book by the same title. The movie is available on the web at

GeneticRouletteMovie.com

NOTE 1:   Organic products are not intentionally genetically modified.

NOTE 2:   Everything said above also applies to corn by-products plus soy and its by-products.

Appendix: Grocery List

Buy fresh and organic whenever possible.

Fruit	Salad	Legumes	Vegetables	Nuts, Raw
Apple *	Avocado @	Beans, dried *	Acorn squash	Almonds * @
Cantaloupe *	Bell peppers	Chickpeas *	Asparagus	Brazil nuts @
Honeydew *	Carrots	Lentils *	Broccoli *	Walnuts @
Kiwi *	Celery *	Lima beans *	Eggplant	
Orange *	Cucumber	Peas, fresh *	Green beans	
	Kale *	Split peas *	Spaghetti Squash	
	Lettuce *		String beans	
	Pepperoncini		Sugar snap peas	
	Spinach *		Sweet potatoes *	
	Sprouts			

Grains	Liquids	Seeds	Meals
Amaranth	Apple juice	Chia	Amy's (no cheese) dinners
Barley	Carrot juice	Flax (ground)	Grits #
Millet	Distilled H_2O	Hemp	Japanese vegetable makkis
Quinoa	Oat milk	Pine nuts	Oatmeal
Rice, brown	Orange juice	Pumpkin	Roasted vegetables
	Rice milk	Sesame *	Soup
		Sunflower	Steamed vegetables

Other	Herbs	Condiments	Supplements
Bread, sprouted	Basil	Bragg Liquid Protein	Kelp (iodine) *
Herbal teas	Cinnamon	Honey	Probiotics
Shredded wheat	Garlic	Iodized sea salt	Vitamin B12
Vegetable broth	Ginger	Pepper	Vitamin D_2
	Parsley	Poultry seasoning	

*   These foods contain helpful alkaline elements.

@ This food is high in fats so use sparingly. Heart disease patients should avoid them.

\# WARNING: In the United States, this food may be genetically modified because it is corn.

Appendix: ACID Food Chart

These foods should be 30% or less of daily intake.

Apricot	Coffee	Molasses	Red Currant
Banana, Ripe	Cranberry	Mustard	Rice
Barley	Currant	Oats	Squash, winter
Barley Malt Syrup	Date	Orange	Strawberry
Beet Sugar	Grains	Papaya	Sunflower seeds
Black Currant	Grapes	Pasta	Tangerine
Blueberry	Grapefruit	Peach	Tea (Black)
Brown Rice	Hazelnuts	Peanut	Vinegar
Brown Rice Syrup	Honey	Pear	Walnuts
Cantaloupe	Italian Plum	Peas	Watermelon
Carob	Lentils	Pistachios	Wheat
Cashews	Macadamia Nuts	Plums *	White Sugar
Cherry, Sweet	Mandarin Orange	Prunes *	Wine
Chocolate	Mango	Raspberry	

* These foods are alkali-producing but have an acidifying effect on the body.

The following foods are neutral but have an acidifying effect on the body.

- Corn oil
- Corn syrup
- Sugar
- Olive oil

Appendix: ALKALINE Food Chart

These foods should be 70% or more of daily intake.

Alfalfa grass	Celery	Lettuce	Raisins
Almonds (sparingly)	Chard	Lima beans	Raspberries
Apples	Cherries, sour	Limes	Rhubarb *
Apricots	Chives	Millet	Rutabaga
Asparagus	Coconut	Molasses	Sauerkraut *
Avocado (fat+protein)	Cucumber	Mushrooms	Sesame seeds
Bananas	Dates, dried	Muskmelon	Soy *
Beans, dried	Fig, dried	Onions	Spelt
Beet greens	Flax seeds	Oranges	Spinach
Beets	Garlic	Parsnips	Strawberries
Blackberries	Grapes	Peaches	Sunflower seeds
Brazil nuts (sparingly)	Green beans	Pears	Tangerines
Broccoli	Hemp seeds	Peas	Tofu *
Brussels sprouts	Kohlrabi	Pineapple	Tomatoes
Cabbage	Leeks (bulbs)	Potatoes	Turnip
Carrot	Lemons	Pumpkin seeds	Watermelon
Cauliflower	Lentils	Radish	Zucchini

* Not recommended—These are alkaline, however they have other properties that are detrimental to the body.

If you have questions, communicate with us via the Contact Us web page of the website below. Please place 'AHS Arthritis Workbook' on the subject line.

www.AHealthSystem.com

A Healing System

Quiz

Workbook

Introduction

Two groups should read this workbook.

1. Health conscious people, their support groups, caregivers and cooks, who are interested in testing their knowledge of the information described in *A HEALING SYSTEM*.

2. Educators who wish to include the healing 'System', or portions thereof, in their training classes.

As a companion to the book *A HEALING SYSTEM*, this workbook provides educators, students of health, and interested readers with:

*   A means of testing and growing their knowledge of the information described in the book *A HEALING SYSTEM.*

*   A starting place for educators wishing to build the system into their teaching programs.

The quiz questions are grouped by category. The questions are intended to be simple, with no tricks.

Quizzes

This workbook exists to enhance your health knowledge base. If you are reading it, then you should have first completed a thorough study of *A Healing System* and fully grasped the concepts presented therein.

The quizzes presented below are open-book tests, if you wish. They will ensure familiarization with all key concepts plus your ability to understand and use the charts and tables in *A Healing System*.

The more you know, the easier it will be to implement the system or any potential subset.

Good luck.

A—Daily PH balancing

1) What causes normally alkaline liver bile to become acidic in the gallbladder?

_____

2) Why should everyone do pH balancing?

_____

3) How much acid ash is acceptable per day?   _____

4) Is a pH of 6.7 alkaline?   Yes / No

5) The digestive track wants to be acidic?   True / False

6) Sugar leaves an alkaline ash.   True / False

7) Coffee leaves an acidic ash.   True / False

8) Brazil nuts leave an alkaline ash.   True / False

9) Raw tomatoes leave what type of ash?   Acid / Alkaline

10) Lemons leave what type of ash?   Acid / Alkaline

B—pH Food Identification

1) List two protein foods that are alkaline ash. _____ , _____

2) When filling in the blanks in this quiz, try to choose those foods you like.

Alkaline ash Protein 1st choice _____

Alkaline ash Protein 2nd choice _____

Alkaline ash Fruit 1 _____

Alkaline ash Fruit 2 _____

Alkaline ash Vegetable 1 _____

Alkaline ash Vegetable 2 _____

Alkaline ash Vegetable 3 _____

Acid ash Protein 1 _____

Acid ash Protein 2 _____

Acid ash Fruit 1 _____

Acid ash Fruit 2 _____

Acid ash Vegetable 1 _____

Acid ash Vegetable 2 _____

C—Food Combining

1) What is the name of the food combining science? _____

2) What are the two inappropriate food combinations associated with the Standard American Diet (SAD)?

a. _____

b. _____

3) Does steak go with potatoes?   Yes / No

4) Avocados go with what foods? _____

5) Melons combine well with what other foods? _____

6) Vegetables do not go well with which foods? _____

7) Cereal and milk go well together.   True / False

8) Protein and carbohydrates go well together.   True / False

9) Carbohydrates and dairy do not go well together.   True / False

10) Citrus can be eaten with anything.   True / False

D—Food Preparation

1) Overcooking your food is acceptable.   True / False

2) Undercooking your food is acceptable.   True / False

3) It is acceptable to cook with which type of oil? _____

4) How should cancer patients prepare raw food? _____

E— Acceptable Foods

1) Yogurt   True / False

2) Desserts   True / False

3) Iodized sea salt   True / False

4) Spices   True / False

5) Foods fried in oil   True / False

6) Vinegar and oil if kept light   True / False

7) Tofu if cooked in water   True / False

F—Drink

1) Drink one half a cup of water per hour.   True / False

2) Drink a cup of tea with each meal.   True / False

3) Lemonade with honey.   True / False

4) Ice water.   True / False

5) One glass of wine per day.   True / False

6) Distilled water is acceptable.   True / False

7) Water is best at what temperature?   _____

8) Drink water 5 minutes before each meal.   True / False

G—Exercise

1) Exercise right before or right after a meal.   Before / After / Neither

2) If exercising is too uncomfortable, quit for a while.   True / False

3) Severity of disease does not affect exercise amount.   True / False

4) Exercise can keep us flexible.   True / False

5) Flexibility is helpful.   True / False

6) All exercise is eustress.   True / False

7) Exercise reduces lymphatic fluid movement   True / False

8) Breathe deeply because... _____

9) Beginners should jump right in to an exercise regimen.   True / False

10) What is eustress? _____

11) Wait ten minutes after a meal before exercising.   True / False

H—Eat Healthy

1) What health problem did cardiologist Robert A. Vogel identify that could happen in a single meal?

_____

_____

_____

2) What are some of the characteristics of a healthy diet?

_____

_____

_____

3) What reasons do people use to select their daily food?

    1. _____

    2. _____

    3. _____

    4. _____

    5. _____

    6. _____

4) Name four healthy foods from the list provided in *A HEALING SYSTEM*.

    1. _____

    2. _____

    3. _____

    4. _____

I—Unhealthy Foods

1) Name the three most mucus forming foods in order, the most severe first.

    1. _____

    2. _____

    3. _____

2) Name some of the grocery-store aisles best avoided during the healing process.

    1. _____

    2. _____

    3. _____

    4. _____

    5. _____

    6. _____

J—Meals

1) List three acceptable meals—at least two foods each—which meet both the pH and food combining requirements.

    1. _____

    2. _____

    3. _____

2) Define mono-meal.

_____

K—Timing: Exercise and Meals

1) What is an acceptable time between meals?

_____

2) What is an acceptable time between meals and exercise?

_____

3) What is an acceptable time between exercise and meals?

_____

L—Water

1) What is the quantity and frequency of water that the average person should drink each day?

_____

2) What is the ideal time between a drink and a meal? _____

M—Nutrition

1) Name five nutrients important to a nutritious diet?

    1. _____

    2. _____

    3. _____

    4. _____

    5. _____

N—Healing

1) Name four things that can be optimized for healing.

    1. _____

    2. _____

    3. _____

    4. _____

2) List 6 things to check into if you are not healing.

1. _____

2. _____

3. _____

4. _____

5. _____

6. _____

O—Testimonials

1. Why are testimonials questionable sources of a successful cure?

_____

_____

2. When are testimonials worth considering?

_____

_____

P—Placebo and Nocebo

1. Define placebo effect.

_____

_____

2. Define nocebo effect.

_____

_____

3. What percentage of drug-trial patients must be excluded because of the placebo and nocebo effects? Give the percentage for each and the total?

_____

4. On average, what percentage of patients are **not** affected by the placebo and nocebo effects? Is it more or less than half?

_____

Q—Healing Keys

1. Name ten keys to healing.

1. _____

2. _____

3. _____

4. _____

5. _____

6. _____

7. _____

8. _____

9. _____

10. _____

R—Reference Material

1. Name two health related movies that have companion books with the same title.

1. _____

2. _____

2. What is the name of the book that identified the healthiest diet by examining the lives of approximately one hundred thousand people? Who are the co-authors?

Title: _____

Authors: _____

3. What book describes a clinical trial of a disease where all patients improved their health, even though some of them were only given months to live? Who is the author?

Title: _____

Author: _____

4. Which cardiologist demonstrated the damage one fatty meal can do to arteries? In the case he presented, how long was the recovery time?

Name: _____

Time: _____

If you have questions, communicate with us via the Contact Us web page of the website below. Please place 'AHS Quiz Workbook' on the subject line.

www.AHealthSystem.com

www.ingramcontent.com/pod-product-compliance
Lightning Source LLC
Chambersburg PA
CBHW080433290526
45791CB00008BA/2475